Dr. Samuel Richard

Benefit of eating fruits

Health benefits of fruits

This book was professionally typeset on Reedsy
Find out more at reedsy.com

Contents

1

INTRODUCTION

Natural products are significant wellsprings of nutrients and carbs like fiber and sugar. They are low in calories and normally sweet. Products of the soil juices are great wellsprings of water, as well. Various natural products contain various nutrients, so eating different fruits is significant. Mangoes, papayas, melons and citrus organic products, similar to oranges and grapefruit, are high in L-ascorbic acid. Melon, apricots, peaches, and nectarines are wellsprings of vitamin A. Entire natural products like apples and grapes contain more fiber than natural product squeezes and sauces, similar to fruit purée and grape juice. Dried natural products like figs, prunes and raisins are great wellsprings of fiber, as well. Canned organic products stuffed in syrup have a great deal of added sugar. They are higher in calories than new natural products. At the point when you search for canned natural products, search for natural product that is stuffed in juice rather than syrup.

2

ADVANTAGES OF EATING LEAFY FRUITS

You have in all likelihood heard for your entire life that you ought to eat your foods grown from the ground. Throughout the long term, it has been demonstrated that having different foods grown from the ground in your eating regimen is very valuable to your well-being .

As per the Habitats for Infectious prevention and Anticipation, just 1 out of 10 grown-ups eat the suggested measure of leafy foods Nonetheless, when you consistently eat products of the soil, you devour the nutrients and minerals that assist your body with working properly.

June is Public New Leafy foods Month, and we're sharing the significance of natural products, vegetables, and how you should rest assured you're getting the right supplements.

Medical advantages of Leafy foods

Leafy foods are advantageous to your body, containing various supplements that have an effect on your well-being .

Here are a few different ways products of the soil benefit your well-being and prosperity.

Supplements

Leafy foods are a decent wellspring of supplements, containing:

1. Nutrients - There are a wide range of nutrients in foods grown from the ground, like nutrients A, C, and E. Nutrients assist with supporting the safe framework, convert food into energy, and that's only the tip of the iceberg.
2. Minerals - Minerals are fundamental in the body and help in making chemicals, as well as supporting the working of the heart and cerebrum.
3. Magnesium - Magnesium manages glucose levels, nerve capability, and that's only the tip of the iceberg.
4. Zinc - Zinc assists the invulnerable framework with fending off microbes.

Leafy foods contain numerous cell reinforcements. They can likewise be mitigating, meaning they battle ongoing irritation that is connected to significant infections like malignant growth and diabetes.

Another fascinating wholesome reality is that various shades of foods grown from the ground address an alternate phytochemical, a compound and supplement delivered by plants.

The shade of a natural product or vegetable likewise shows what sort of supplements it has. Red foods grown from the ground contain potassium and L-ascorbic acid, though orange and yellow products of the soil are high in fiber.

Other Medical advantages

Eating products of the soil can assist you with dealing with your weight since they are low in calories and high in water content. These elements make foods grown from the ground an extraordinary choice for a feast or tidbit.

Leafy foods likewise contain fiber and water, which can assist with keeping you full and fulfilled longer. This will assist with keeping you from eating carelessly over the course of the day.

Eating foods grown from the ground gives you supplements, yet with enduring medical advantages too. Leafy foods can assist with bringing down your gamble of hypertension, diabetes, weight, and heart disease. With regards to picking and eating products of the soil, there are some do's and don't. Here are a few hints on picking the best produce.

1. **Get it. In the event that a natural product or vegetable is delicate when you realize it shouldn't be, like a banana or avocado, try not to get it. There's a decent opportunity it's over-ready or wounded.**

2. **Pick what's in season. Leafy foods taste best when they're in-season. For instance, strawberries are best in the mid year. Watermelon is likewise best throughout the mid year months, which is extraordinary an extraordinary nibble since it contains a lot of water and helps in hydration.**

Keep leafy foods new. Leafy foods can endure longer whenever dealt with and put away appropriately. Here are a few hints to keep your leafy foods new.

1. **Wash and dry. Wash your products of the soil, ideally with a foods grown from the ground wash, then ensure they are dry prior to putting away.**

2. **Refrigerate matured organic product. Most natural product ages at room temperature. Whenever it's matured, you can put in the refrigerator to stop the maturing system, which will assist it with enduring a couple of days longer.**

3. **Freeze. A few leafy foods can be frozen up to three months. Once frozen, these products of the soil can be utilized in smoothies or defrosted and utilized in various recipes.**

Eat More Leafy foods

Leafy foods can be eaten new, cooked, frozen, canned, or dried, which gives you a lot of choices with regards to adding them to your dinners.

Here are a few thoughts on how you can consolidate different leafy foods in your eating regimen.

1. **Cook vegetables to go with your supper. The choices to add vegetables to your supper are perpetual. Take a stab at baking a yam, steaming broccoli, or barbecuing asparagus. On the off chance that you need a more straightforward choice, have a go at cutting up the**

entirety of your vegetables and broiling them generally on a similar sheet container.

2. Utilize frozen products of the soil in a smoothie. This is an incredible method for getting supplements while partaking in a virus treat. Smoothies are likewise kind with the stomach related framework in view of the consistency. You can likewise add yogurt or a nut margarine on the off chance that you could do without the flavor of the foods grown from the ground alone.

3. Eat new or dried natural product as a bite. If you would rather not get ready new natural product nor have a method for keeping it cold, attempt dried natural product. Dried natural product is not difficult to take with you anyplace and can be added to snacks like yogurt or granola.

3

ADVANTAGES OF EATING ORGANIC PRODUCTS AROUND EVENING TIME

On the off chance that you're having organic products for supper, eat just natural products. Different sorts of food, notwithstanding natural products, may cause heartburn. Natural product assimilation is totally unique in relation to that of other nutrition classes. Thus, in the event that you're having a light supper with different kinds of food, stand by 30 minutes prior to eating organic product. More natural products with some light food are not suggested. Likewise, while eating natural products around evening time, keep away from natural products that are excessively sweet or excessively harsh.

Try not to hit the sack following eating organic products:

Organic products are dependably advantageous in light of the fact that they are high in fiber. While eating natural products, the key is to eat just natural products. If you have any desire to eat natural product with or after a feast, ensure you eat it inside thirty minutes. It isn't prescribed to eat two kinds of food simultaneously in light of the fact that our bodies digest various sorts of food at various rates. At the point when you eat organic products just after a dinner, the natural products digest first.

Additionally, eating organic products just before sleep time might bring about sleep deprivation. At the point when fructose, the sugar in natural products, is consumed by the body, the body encounters a flood of energy. In that state, heading to sleep following eating natural products might cause sleep deprivation. It is best not to head to sleep following eating some natural product. Organic products contain more sugar than the other nutrition classes joined. To have just organic products for supper, that is fine. Simply make sure to hit the sack thirty minutes after the fact.

More organic products in the nights are great, particularly for those experiencing corpulence, lack of sleep, blockage, hypertension, and different circumstances. Pick organic products that are less prepared. Organic products that are in season can be eaten, for example, banana assortments that are not excessively sharp, ready mangoes that are less sweet, apples, papaya, guava, watermelon, mythical serpent organic product, etc. The key is to stay away from incredibly sweet or tart natural products. The people who have recently had a stroke can likewise eat organic products that are high in fiber and low in pleasantness and sharpness between feasts.

Any natural product, like an apple or guava, ought to be eaten entire as opposed to stripped prior to eating. A natural product just eating routine for supper is incredibly helpful. The individuals who are blocked up or overweight, notwithstanding, should practice alert. Others can have a light supper of two chapattis followed by a little bowl of organic product following 60 minutes. Ensure you hit the sack no less than 30 minutes in the wake of eating organic product. Natural products best taking for supper

Kiwi organic product

You could realize that these green, sweet little organic products work out positively in a natural product salad, yet you probably won't realize that they could likewise assist you with having a more serene rest. In a review featured by College of North Carolina at Sanctuary Slope, the utilization of two kiwifruits in something like one hour of sleep time could diminish mid-rest attentiveness by an astounding 30 percent. On the off chance that you really can't stay unconscious as the night progressed, take a stab at adding kiwi organic product to your shopping list.

Bananas

Despite the fact that you could as a rule have bananas with breakfast, they really contain elevated degrees of potassium and magnesium, regular muscle relaxers that can permit your body to feel more quiet and prepared for rest. Likewise, the sugars in bananas can expand your lethargy. So on the off chance that you're feeling somewhat peckish before bed, feel free to strip your direction to a superior night's rest.

Cherries and cherry juice contain elevated degrees of melatonin, a chemical in the cerebrum that controls your rest guideline. One concentrate even demonstrates the way that drinking tart cherry juice could further develop stay in bed individuals who experience the ill effects of a sleeping disorder. Led by Louisiana State College, the investigation discovered that grown-ups who polished off only 8 ounces of tart cherry squeeze two times each day rested for 85 extra minutes.

Berries including blueberries, raspberries and blackberries contain extremely elevated degrees of cell reinforcements. As per specialists at the Public Rest Establishment, cell reinforcements can shield you from the pressure of a rest problem, which can cause oxidation in the body. Consuming cell reinforcement rich berries before bed can assist with lessening your generally actual pressure, consequently permitting you to have a more soothing rest.

Pineapple

One more fruity treat to appreciate before bed is the modest pineapple. Likewise high in melatonin, specialists found that subsequent to eating pineapple, the melatonin markers in the body could increment by 266%. This implies that consistently consuming this sweet treat before bed could assist you with nodding off quick and stay unconscious longer.

4

ADVANTAGES OF EATING ORGANIC PRODUCTS DURING PREGNANCY

When pregnant, ladies need to eat thc right food so their children can get the supplements expected to go through the necessary physiological changes in uteri. Concentrates on show that babies that don't get legitimate sustenance from the beginning are inclined to sicknesses further down the road.

Eating organic products during pregnancy has a few advantages for both mother and child. First of all, organic products are supplement thick, loaded with nutrients, minerals, and fiber. Eating an eating routine comprising of a blend of organic products gives you and your child the vast majority of the significant supplements.

Look at This Rundown of Best Natural products For Pregnant Ladies!

1. Guava

Guava contains various supplements and is in this way one of the most outstanding organic products to eat during pregnancy. It is protected to eat all through pregnancy, loosening up muscles and help absorption. Guava is wealthy in fiber, which beefs up food and keeps you feeling full, help solid discharge forestalls clogging and hemorrhoids. Keep away from voraciously consuming food guava and consistently eat ready ones during pregnancy.

2. Banana

One more organic product high in dietary fiber is banana! Aside from this, bananas are loaded with fundamental unsaturated fats like omega-3 and omega-6. Omega-3 unsaturated fats bring down the gamble of per-term work and conveyance, toxemia, wretchedness, and help in expanding birth weight. Omega-6 unsaturated fats are fundamental for heart well being.

Bananas are additionally loaded with significant nutrients like B-intricate and C, minerals like magnesium, manganese, copper, and selenium, making them the best natural products to eat during pregnancy. Potassium in banana reduces liquid maintenance, balances electrolytes, and lifts the resistant framework.

3.Orange

Orange and other citrus organic products have L-ascorbic acid in overflow. This nutrient is pivotal for the development and advancement of the child's bones and teeth. L-ascorbic acid additionally ingests iron, which is a critical mineral for the body.

In particular, L-ascorbic acid is a cell reinforcement, decreasing harm brought about by free revolutionaries.

Besides, oranges are a decent wellspring of fiber and folic corrosive. A water-dis solvable B nutrient, folic corrosive forestalls development surrenders connected with the mind and spinal rope in the embryo, so ensure oranges are among the organic products to eat during pregnancy.

4.Apple

Cancer prevention agents and L-ascorbic acid in apples is significant for in general well-being . Apples additionally contain B nutrients, which keep red platelets sound. Concentrates on show that apples bring down the gamble of sensitivities and asthma in youth. Likewise, apples are loaded with iron which helps support hemoglobin creation and forestalls frailty.

5.Kiwi

This wholesome force to be reckoned with is plentiful in dietary fiber, folic corrosive, nutrients C and E, potassium, carotenoids, and cancer prevention agents. Kiwis additionally have a few other minor elements that add to in general well-being for both mother and kid.

6. Apricot

Apricots contain crucial nutrients and minerals like folic corrosive, calcium, potassium, and magnesium. Dried apricots are a rich wellspring of iron and fiber, helping creation of red platelets and controlling stomach related cycles, and consequently are perfect as natural products to eat during pregnancy.

Berries

Strawberries, raspberries, blueberries, and more are loaded with L-ascorbic acid, folic corrosive, beta carotene, cancer prevention agents, potassium, and that's just the beginning. These assistance to fabricate the child's body and resistant framework.

5

ADVANTAGES OF EATING ORGANIC FRUITS DAY TO DAY

Eating organic product gives medical advantages — individuals who eat more foods grown from the ground as a feature of a generally speaking solid eating regimen are probably going to have a decreased gamble of a few ongoing illnesses. Natural products give supplements indispensable to well-being and support of your body. As a feature of an in general solid eating regimen, eating food varieties, for example, natural products that are lower in calories per cup rather than some other more unhealthy food might be valuable in assisting with bringing down calorie consumption. Eating an eating routine wealthy in vegetables and natural products as a component of a generally solid eating regimen might decrease risk for coronary illness, including cardiovascular failure and stroke. Eating an eating routine wealthy in certain vegetables and organic products as a feature of a by and large sound eating routine might safeguard against specific kinds of malignant growths.

Adding organic product can assist with expanding admission of fiber and potassium which are significant supplements that numerous Americans don't get enough of in their eating regimen. New organic products are normally sweet and pack colossal healthful advantages also. Organic products go about as cleaning agents for your body, give you energy and supply a huge range of nutrients, minerals and cell reinforcements that advance great well-being . Organic product may likewise advance the solid flow of your blood, which additionally diminishes your gamble of coronary illness. Willett adds that citrus natural products, like oranges and grapefruit, might be especially advantageous at decreasing your gamble of coronary illness.

Adding a few servings of organic product to your day to day diet might diminish your possibilities creating esophageal, stomach and cellular breakdown in the lungs. You may likewise have the option to decrease your gamble of mouth, throat, ovarian, bladder and colon disease. Lower hazard of brain tube abandons: Folate (folic corrosive) assists the body with framing red platelets. Ladies of childbearing age who might become pregnant and those in the main trimester of pregnancy need sufficient folate. Folate forestalls brain tube birth deformities, for example, spinabifida. Assurance against cell harm: An eating design where natural product is essential for a generally sound eating routine gives cancer prevention agents that assist with fixing harm done by free extremists and may safeguard against specific tumors. It might likewise emphatically affect stomach related well-being . Polyphenols are cancer prevention agents that have been displayed to adjust stomach micro ecology , or the extent of sound versus unsafe microbes.

6

ADVANTAGES OF EATING NATURAL PRODUCTS FOR THE SKIN

Organic products can be beneficial for your skin. There are different advantages of organic products for the skin that you can benefit of by basically integrating them into your day to day daily practice. Loaded with fundamental nutrients and minerals, they can work a wide range of miracles for your skin and assist you with putting your best face forward. Enjoying an organic product rich eating routine will give you various medical advantages and work on your skin from the back to front. These delicious treats can likewise be utilized topically to treat your skin worries for faster outcomes. Organic product removes are utilized in numerous restorative details, as well, as their advantages are really worth collecting for excellence purposes. L-ascorbic acid is vital for a solid body. It reinforces resistance for inside well-being as well as lifts collagen creation in the body, subsequently further developing the skin's obstruction capabilities for outer well-being and magnificence. It is the fixing you really want to load up on day to day as your body can't normally deliver L-ascorbic acid, nor does it hold it inside your blood for sometime in the future. In the event that you're hoping to get in on its advantages for sparkling skin, consume organic products that are plentiful in the nutrient, for example, citrus organic products consistently. Such natural products are likewise awesome to battle skin inflammation. Think organic products like oranges, grapefruits, and pineapples.

Tip: To treat unexpected breakouts, dunk a small cotton ball in pineapple squeeze, and tape it to the skin inflammation sore. Require this off following 30 minutes, and wash with cool water. Berries have a high cell reinforcement limit that helps the skin. The polyphenols that are found in berries assist with safeguarding skin from natural aggressors and different indications of maturing. Berries are perfect for effective utilization as well. They can be squashed and used to cause normal cleans as they to have shedding properties. Organic products like strawberries are additionally rich in salicylic corrosive, which can assist with peeling skin break out causing microbes. In the event that you are utilizing berries on your skin, it is critical to initially lead a fix test. Tip: Cut up a strawberry, and tenderly rub it on the skin to shed and keep skin break out under control. Clean up after with cool water.

Tropical natural products have various skin-spoiling benefits; they accompany fundamental nutrients and saturating properties. These natural products can be applied straightforwardly to skin. Tropical organic products, for example, papayas and bananas are particularly astounding for feeding the skin and offering skin-lighting up properties. Both of these organic products are plentiful in potassium and vitamin A. Papain, a functioning compound found in papaya, sheds dead skin cells when applied to skin.

Tip: Rub papaya strips on your skin and allow them to sit for 20 minutes. Wash off with water. This will likewise hydrate your skin and light up your complexion.

Your skin is the biggest organ of your body. To keep it sound, it is vital to guarantee you are eating the right food sources, regardless of whether you use skincare items topically. Organic products are normally low in fat and calories, and you don't need to stress over cholesterol with regards to this nutrition class. Organic products are great wellsprings of fundamental supplements that your body needs however doesn't necessarily get enough of, like potassium, dietary filaments, L-ascorbic acid, and folic corrosive. These supplements help physical processes that advance skin well-being and lift cell recovery.

Tip: Consume a rainbow of natural products consistently to get sparkling skin.

At the point when you decide to topically apply organic products to your skin, you are harvesting their integrity for your skin straightforwardly, and that implies faster outcomes. Beside consuming natural products for sound skin, applying them topically permits your skin to straightforwardly take in the supplements they bring to the table. Normal oils from organic products can help the skin when applied topically, and skin illnesses like skin break out, dim spots, and discoloration can be dealt with all the more actually as the effective application gives designated activity.

Tip: Cut and hold the strips and skins from the natural products that you eat, and apply them to your skin. Wash off with cool water following 15 minutes.

You can without much of a stretch lift your day to day nutrient admission by drinking custom made juices. Green juices are a decent decision as you can expand the impacts of your natural products alongside vegetables. Consolidate natural products with vegetables and you might in fact include a touch of flavor along with the remaining blend to make yummy juices to drink consistently. Attempt a green juice made with kale, pineapple and cucumber, which will offer you every one of the nutrients you really want consistently.

Tip: Consider delicious vegetables that can be changed over into juice, and afterward add natural products to support the flavor. Try not to add sugar to these juices.

7

COULD EATING AN EXCESSIVE AMOUNT OF NATURAL PRODUCT BE TERRIBLE FOR YOU?

Natural product is a vital piece of a smart dieting plan. Organic products contain numerous supplements that your body needs. As a matter of fact, a solid eating routine that incorporates natural product has been found to diminish your gamble of a few constant infections.

Yet, organic product contains regular sugars, and a few kinds are genuinely high in calories. So certain individuals might keep thinking about whether they're eating a lot of it.

There's nothing that you can't eat a lot of. Yet, truly it's difficult to get an excessive amount of natural product. Most Americans don't eat enough of it, as a matter of fact. Grown-ups ought to eat somewhere around 1 ½ cups of organic product consistently.

Nonetheless, a "fruitarian" diet, in which you eat barely anything yet natural product, can hold you back from getting an adequate number of supplements from different food sources. Specialists suggest that 25%-30% of your eating routine be comprised of organic product.

Also, shouldn't something be said about the sugar in organic product? The sugar you ought to stress over, specialists say, is the additional sort you track down in soft drinks, treats, and numerous different items. Since organic product contains fiber, your body responds diversely to its normal sugars.

All things considered, on the off chance that you eat enormous bits, an excess of natural product sugar could add to medical issues, for example,

1. Weight gain
2. Diabetes
3. Inconveniences with pancreatic and kidney conditions
4. Tooth rot
5. Lacks of vitamin B12, calcium, vitamin D, and omega-3 unsaturated fats

On the off chance that you're attempting to get thinner, eating a great deal of organic product can disrupt your endeavors. While carbohydrate levels are unassuming in many sorts of new natural product, they can soar on the off chance that you're tasting a ton of natural product juice, making smoothies (which can amount to 300 calories or more) or drinking a ton of dried natural products, which are a wellspring of concentrated sugar. Individuals who eat a ton of natural product are many times well-being and weight-cognizant yet can't comprehend the reason why they're not losing pounds. Eating an excessive amount of natural product can likewise raise your serum fatty substances, which can increment cardiovascular gamble. The high glycemic heap of certain types of natural product can incite insulin obstruction and demolish metabolic condition. Individuals with this issue are encouraged to eat just entire foods grown from the ground servings of dried organic products to one-quarter cup each day. Assuming that you eat canned organic products, pick water-stuffed items and channel them prior to serving.

Despite the fact that it is undeniably challenging to eat an excess of organic product, it can work out. In the event that this occurs, the negative aftereffects will generally be connected with assimilation in light of natural product's high fiber content. "Gambles related with overabundance natural product admission incorporate stomach uneasiness, looseness of the bowels, bulging, acid reflux, and likely supplement lacks on the off chance that abundance natural product is supplanting other significant supplements in the eating regimen.

Organic product is a significant piece of a solid eating regimen, yet did you realize you can really eat excessively? It's valid, eating a lot of organic product can really expand your gamble for coronary episode and diabetes, and damage your weight reduction objectives. It can likewise cause a large group of different issues like tooth rot.

At the point when you eat an excessive amount of organic product, you can raise your degrees of serum fatty substances, which add to cardiovascular breakdown and respiratory failures. On the off chance that you're in danger for this, eating a ton of organic product can exacerbate it. Elevated degrees of fructose have likewise been connected to causing irritation, raising circulatory strain and harming your kidneys. Another outcome is insulin opposition, so in the event that you're on the edge of getting diabetes, or have diabetes, a great deal of natural product can exacerbate it.

8

BENEFIT OF CONSUMING FRUITS BEFORE MEAL

Consuming natural products is significant in adjusted and solid eating routine. Products of the soil oblige in the primary layer of food pyramid as recommended by Service of Well-being. This implies products of the soil should be consumed in rather enormous sum for example 3 servings for vegetables and 2 servings for natural products in a day. When is the best opportunity to consume organic products?

Overall organic products can be consumed at whenever of the day. Nonetheless, specialists propose of consuming natural products best in the first part of the day and as in the middle between feasts. Natural products can likewise be consumed as a hors d'oeuvre prior to having a genuine legitimate feast. This is gainful particularly in the event that somebody is on a tight eating routine program to shed pounds. Natural products contain high fiber consequently bringing about sluggish absorption cycle and making somebody feel full for delayed time. This will lessen the individual calorie consumption during their genuine feast.

Natural products contain and wealthy in cell reinforcements. They are fundamental regular wellsprings of cell reinforcements. By consuming natural products, these cell reinforcements help to kill free revolutionaries which are unsafe to cells which can prompt different diseases including malignant growth.

Consuming organic products before dinner likewise guarantees a superior retention of supplements. Organic products contain sugar that calls for a delayed investment to be processed and retained. Consequently whenever contrasted with having organic products after a feast the supplements from natural products are better processed and ingested if having them before a dinner.

Illustration of natural products that wealthy in fiber including apple, pear, banana and raspberry and illustration of organic products that wealthy in cancer prevention agent including grapes, strawberry and papaya. For diabetic patients the admission of organic products is prompted not to be in that frame of mind to keep away from the abundance sugar.

Its an obvious fact that smart dieting implies expanding your admission of leafy foods. As simple as this might sound, incorporating it tends to be troublesome. Grown-ups will generally eat not exactly the suggested measures of fundamental supplements, including organic products

Eating natural product before a feast not just empowers additional organic product consumption, it might likewise assist you with controlling your weight and meet your nutrient and mineral necessities.

Eating a piece of organic product just before your feast might assist with controlling your eating during supper time. Plunking down for a dinner while you're starving can prompt gorging and extreme calorie consumption. Eating a piece of organic product before a feast permits you to put something low calorie into your stomach. Natural products are viewed as a low-energy-thickness food. This implies that they give a limited quantity of energy, or calories, for a high volume. Eating low-energy-thickness food sources, particularly before a dinner, assists with diminishing your generally speaking caloric admission, which fits weight control.

Eating organic product before a dinner builds your admission of fiber for that feast, on the grounds that most natural product is high in fiber. At the point when you eat fiber, you feel more full for a more extended time frame in light of the fact that fiber dials back processing. It additionally assists block the assimilation of fats and cholesterol, making your feast that much with bettering for you. On the off chance that you are diabetic, fiber in your feast implies more slow processing and a more slow arrival of glucose into your circulatory system. At the point when this happens, your glucose is better controlled. High-fiber organic product sources remember apples and pears with the skin for, raspberries and bananas.

9

CONCLUSION

Help yourself out and eat your natural products. They are totally a significant piece of having a fair supplement thick eating regimen. It truly is an injury to disparage organic product like some trend slims down have done in light of the fact that it makes individuals reluctant to eat something so nutritious. So my companions, eat your leafy foods blissful.